CREATIVE CHILDBIRTH

*The Leclaire Method of Easy Birthing
Through
Hypnosis and Rational-Intuitive Thought*

Michelle Leclaire O'Neill, Ph.D., R.N.

Papyrus

Creative Childbirth
A Papyrus Book 1993

ISBN #0-9633087-3-4
Library of Congress Catalogue Number 92081691

Cover by: Francesca Bianchi Design
Artwork and Layout: Francesca Bianchi Design

*Dedicated to the women of Our Lady of the Angels
and Saint John's Parish, Bronx, New york City*

Eugenia Persico-Leclaire, mother of 9
Lorraine O'Neill, mother of 10

Mrs. Sweeney, mother of 5
Josie Smith, mother of 5
Grace Singleton, mother of 12
Agnes McKee, mother of 7
Mrs. Monahan, mother of 10
Mrs. Ganly, mother of 5
Marguerite Schaffer Balestrieri, mother of 11
Mrs. Gorman, mother of 6
Margie Callanan, mother of 6
Rita Cawley, mother of 6
Mrs. Robinson, mother of 6
Rita Murray, mother of 5
Gert Casey, mother of 4
Norma Joyce, mother of 4
Nora Martin Boland, mother of 3
Grace O'Neill-McHugh, mother of 1
Mrs. Green, mother of 3
Mrs. Martin, mother of 2
Mrs. Weaver, mother of 3
Mrs. Ferrari, mother of 2
Mrs. Ward, mother of 3
Margaret Persico Erhardt, mother of 4

◈ CONTENTS

▓ Introduction

Growing up as the eldest of nine children, in an Irish Catholic New York neighborhood, birthing was both an everyday event and a joyous and sacred occasion. When I recall the conversations I heard about childbirth I do not remember stories of pain and long, hard labors, but rather of how much faster this one was than the one before. Recognition and respect were bestowed upon the women with the greatest number of children. Babies were so very special that an entire room in the basement of our grand old apartment building, St. Alban's Court, was designated as a "carriage room."

When I birthed my own babies there was no celebratory environment, just a cold, dark hospital room and a bed with side rails. I don't know how I envisioned all the births that took place in my neighborhood, but it certainly wasn't in the depressing, lonely conditions of a hospital labor room. I think I imagined all the women surrounding the birthing mother and cheering her on. I imagined all the fathers down at the local Irish bar, drinking up a storm while the "pregnant" father paced or twirled anxiously on the bar stool. When the blessed event occurred, a phone call was made to the pub, a cheer ran through the house, a taxi was called, and the proud father and his cronies piled together into the cab for further fanfare as they drove to visit the newborn Pope or Mother Theresa. There was much joy and hope surrounding birthing. A great miracle happened each time a newborn entered the neighborhood, and the excitement was felt and talked about by all.

I loved the feelings engendered by the birthing process as I grew up. It is these feelings of hope and joy that I felt were lacking in childbirth as I experienced it, and in the tales told by friends and clients. Thus, again and again I came back to the women. The Leclaire classes for hypnosis and childbirth then ultimately found their origin in the women of Our Lady of the Angels and St. John's Parish in New York. It is to them that I gratefully dedicate this book.

I have read many books on childbirth, and the only one for me that touches on the miracle and wonder of it all is *Childbirth Without Fear* by Grantly Dick Read, M.D. Dr. Read, as early as the 1920's, realized the importance of an holistic approach to childbirth. He saw the pregnant mother as a human being, and not just as a body in a pregnant state. He realized the importance of an interdisciplinary approach, i.e., that psychology interfaces with sociology and anthropology. He also realized that the woman who is pregnant has been influenced in a complex way by her biology and by her social and cultural environment.

It is from this framework, and from the foundation set before me by the wonderful women educators in the dramatic Ursuline and Sister of Charity garb that the Leclaire method developed. Each agrees that we function as part of a system, both external — such as family, community, society — and internal, such as mind, body and spirit. The Leclaire method sees childbirth as an affirmative acknowledgement of these external and internal systems.

Through childbirth, we can grasp all of our dimensions and expand them to an exciting participation with the life force. Thus, Leclaire deals primarily with how the psychological and cultural mantle of the mother, and her support person, alter the physical process of pregnancy, labour, birthing and all postpartum experience.

Leclaire works primarily with the psychological preparation as a precursor to physiological preparation. I would like to assure you that when your body and mind are in a relaxed state, proper breathing, i.e., breathing that will enhance the baby's progress through the birth canal, will automatically follow.

Mai is a good example of a mother who succeeded with proper psychological preparation. Her doctor could not understand why all of a sudden during the second trimester her pregnancy was threatened. He placed her on bed rest, and I was called to make a home visit. I knew her from the class and enjoyed her playful energy. She is very open, loving, and joyous, and also a high-powered business woman, who took great pride in competing in a predominantly male market-place, and who, more often than not, closed big deals that even the most seasoned male tycoon might find intimidating. Mai saw it as a game; and her playfulness, calculating intelligence, tremendous energy, perseverance, and competitive spirit made her a formidable opponent. She was on the verge of closing two big deals during her fifth month.

Remember, being confined to bed created much anxiety for her. When I walked into her spacious home, I was directed to her office/bedroom. Here she lay, amidst a pile of papers, two telephones, a fax machine, and an at-home foetal monitoring device. She was holding court in her room with her houseman, cook, and maid. She was in high spirits, and seemed to be enjoying it all.

I started to laugh as I said to her, "One quick home visit and your OB would see that there is nothing mysterious about your condition. It is exactly as it should be." Neither her body nor her baby could take the stress of her lifestyle. The job was now to help her align her mind, her body, and her spirit, and to help her to make some realistic choices in eliminating the stress of her lifestyle.

Mai needed to learn how to initiate a union of opposites. Until Mai learned how to deal with the realization that the baby was intruding on her lifestyle, her pregnancy would remain in jeopardy. Once she could accept this and understand her ambivalence about this intrusion, and her psychological rejection of the child, she could eliminate her physical rejection of it. Now she would be able to work at what she wanted to let in and what she wanted to let go. She was able to reconcile her making it in the world with her adaptive feminine receptive rhythm. Being of a pragmatic mind, Mai soon realized what needed to be done, decided to look seriously at the situation at hand, and to resolve it to the best of her ability. I'm happy to say that she held her beautiful baby boy to term and then some. She wouldn't be Mai is she didn't go a bit overboard in one direction or another. She had a C section, and recovered beautifully and rapidly, using all her new techniques to bring her mind and body closer to being of one spirit.

I find it very exciting how our bodies present to us the symbol of what we need to address in our psyches.

The Leclaire method further evolved as a result of working with O. Carl Simonton, M.D., around people with life-threatening illness. Ironically, there was more joy surrounding getting well again, or accepting dying and death as a part of life, than there was around birthing a new life. I came to realize through helping people during the getting-well process, or in helping them prepare for the dying process, that hope was always available to them (hope being a belief that beneficial things are possible). Hope is the belief in options, and hopelessness the belief in no options. Hopelessness is rigid and absolute.

I began to see that the choices surrounding childbirth were limited. As I saw it, there did not seem to be enough room for joy in labour and birthing. There did not seem to be much room for an openness and curiosity to life. I saw a lot of hopelessness, which to me was a signal for a change. I remembered all the wonderful women of Kingsbridge and I wanted to recreate in some fashion the "ode to joy" they so beautifully orchestrated.

There is much preparation that goes into being able to be relaxed enough to participate in the techniques surrounding hypnosis; thus, the book does not begin with hypnosis, but rather ends with it.

The pattern for pregnancy, labour and childbirth is determined by the mother and her support person's usual way of dealing with stress, discomfort, intimacy, involvement and joy. Thus, we must early on intervene to structure healthy belief systems in these areas.

It is necessary that we deal with the myths surrounding childbirth in the twentieth century, and with the feelings and fears, hopes and ambivalences of both the mothers and fathers. The classes are of seven weeks' duration, and this book hopes to deal with the issues that have arisen in the classes — issues that, when cleared from the sensorium, allow a serene mind to remain out of the body's way. Our bodies do know exactly how to birth our babies in a calm, joyous, easy manner. It is we, acting under the manifesto of our culture, who often get in our own way. I do hope you and your support person enjoy the process of preparing for a creative and joyous birthing.

Take time to go through each chapter, paying special attention to the exercises at the end of each chapter. It is better to do one or two or three chapters a week than to try to do them all at once. Here is a suggested schedule:

Week I:
Chapter One —   Taking the initial steps toward integrating attitude and experience.

Chapter Two —   Examination of myths surrounding childbirth.

Week II:
Chapter Three —   Redefinition of labour.

Chapter Four —   The path to the universal truth that lies within each of us.

Chapter Five —   Ego, Instinct, Self and the Dream - the connection between the unconscious and the dilation of the cervix.

Week III:
Chapter Six —   Pain and the psycho-neuro-hormonal connection. Also, a few more myths of our culture that relate to pain in childbirth.

Chapter Seven —   Nutrition and exercise. Learning how to set realistic goals for yourself.

Week IV:
Chapter Eight —   What hypnosis is and isn't. Discussion of preconceived notions about hypnosis.

Chapter Nine —   Hypnosis techniques.

Chapter Ten —   Techniques to Deepen Hypnotic State.

Week V:
Chapter Eleven —   Music and Healing. How specific music engages your concentration and regulates your alpha state.

Chapter Twelve —   Herstory

◆ Chapter One

Integrating Attitude and Experience

Pregnancy is not an illness and not a medical problem. It is a natural state of being, in which it is beneficial for both the father and mother to connect to the nurturing instinct. When the father connects to his male mothering instincts he often finds a new, calmer and richer way of experiencing all areas of his life.

Within the Leclaire method, nurturing/mothering is approached as an integral part of both womanhood and manhood. Alas, the feminine instinct all too often lies dormant in the man. By remaining open and curious during pregnancy and childbirth, men are given a wonderful opportunity to become whole.

Within the medical model the doctor, often a male, delivers the baby, i.e., he takes control of the woman's body and intervenes in some mechanized, technological way. In our rational/intuitive birthing model, the woman, her support person and the baby participate together in the birthing process. If the woman has chosen the proper attendant she/he will cooperate and support the mother's natural birthing process rather than imposing a harried, judgmental, and dictatorial model upon her.

One of the physicians with whom I work is most supportive of her patient's choices. Yvonne Fried, OB, Gyn, M.D., sees her role as unique to the patient she is with. She states:

"To the women in search of mates I am the beholder of confidences, the most far reaching of which is their fear of the AIDS virus. For the woman laden with child I am a trusted transition object. For the woman approaching her late thirties or forties who longs to conceive but has not yet done so, I represent the technological medical hope. In my daily purposeful movements from examining room to examining room I maintain a chameleon-like attention to detail. Without this I would be like every other disinterested, unlistening OB-Gyn who pretends to speak to women about their health care."

Dr. Yvonne Fried's initial interest in hypnosis and the Leclaire method developed out of a need to better understand how verbal and nonverbal communication might improve patient compliance with suggested therapies. Many of Dr. Fried's patients and support people have been through the Leclaire method. Dr. Fried has observed that the most significant difference between this group and the patients who have not been through the classes is in how they are in labour. Dr. Fried states:

"I have even had to restructure how I perceive patients' pain tolerance, progress in labour and how I query patients in labour. Patients who have used Leclaire and hypnosis in labour show none of the somatic and physiological signs of distress that I have seen in patients who have studied Lamaze alone."

To create is to bring into existence or to sustain a life or being. It is through a female and male partnership that new life becomes. To sustain this new life, men and women need to provide nourishment and support through active interest, encouragement, participation, help and cooperation.

The dualistic philosophy that still dominates medical thinking, that holds mind and body as distinct and separate, is an artificial bifurcation. Here in this book we will trace the thread that is woven through the mind/body of the mother and the father to the foetus.

In one of the class sessions, the mother and father are asked to do a crayon drawing; the father is asked to draw his partner's body, their baby, himself, and any external situations that may be interfering with a healthy relationship of the father, the mother and the baby. One father drew himself trying to crawl inside his wife's uterus with the baby. "I want to be safe inside, also," he declared. "He has it made, all curled up in there. I have to worry about being the caretaker of everyone. I wish I could just be curled up inside the safety of the amniotic fluid."

Another father drew himself physically supporting his wife, and then decided this was how he wished he could be, rather than how he was able to be. He then began to discuss his fear of fainting when crowning took place. Through much discussion, a decision was made that he would be his wife's support person up to that point, and then he would leave her with her second support person. After a few private sessions they graciously accepted and understood each other's wishes. Prior to the drawing of the picture this couple had been having increased arguments. After discussing his fears and coming to an agreement, the arguing subsided, and the father was able to return to a nurturing figure. The father who longed to be inside the womb with his baby was, in fact, a very nurturing husband and was also very supportive to the other fathers in the group.

In learning how to integrate attitude and environment we see how pregnancy, labour and birthing can be experienced as an harmonious process, thus becoming one of the greatest opportunities to transcend fear and pain. Through a centered participation in the marvelous miracle of change, growth and life, great joy is available to all.

Leclaire believes in childbirth as an affirmative acknowledgement of womanhood/manhood and as one of the most exciting ways to participate with the life force. The object then is to enable the mother to do the best that she can to use the new information and tools she now has at hand and to move in the direction of a pain-free childbirth. It is during pregnancy that a woman really needs for family to be a priority over both her career and her spouse's career. When a mother is safely able to articulate her desire for more time and attention from her partner, when she is able to deal with these common issues in a group, only to find that she is not alone in her needs, wants and desires, much hurt and pain in the spousal relationship is abandoned. When marital problems are dealt with rather than denied, the mother does not have to cling to her foetus as her only ally in this family. If the father is willing to acknowledge the mother's needs and compromise in some agreeable way, the possibility of a joyous birthing is now closer at hand.

Our task then is to deal with our attitudes and to change them in a way that will help to facilitate a joyous and pain-free birthing. Our task is also to reteach our bodies/our egos that it is helpful to be of "one spirit" — to teach our egos that it is helpful to relinquish our own critical faculties. It is important to learn how to keep the ego out of the way of the work that our bodies/ourselves have done for centuries.

It is the task of this book then to reinforce positive belief systems and to help you redefine your unhealthy belief systems.

How a woman feels about pregnancy and childbirth is a direct correlate to how she will experience pregnancy and childbirth. Thus, it is imperative that the mother learns to deal with her conflicting attitudes about marriage, pregnancy, birthing, motherhood, breast feeding, and her career. These need to be attended to in order to prevent the displacement of these feelings into a physical resistance manifested by anxiety, fear, pain, and even maternal and/or foetal distress. Take a few moments now, if you will, to do the following exercise:

Mother's Exercise

Draw a picture of your body and your baby. Include in this picture anything in your life that you see that might be a source of worry to you, and anything that you feel might be acting as a deterrent to your having the most joyous pregnancy/birthing possible. Do the drawing as quickly and as spontaneously as you can, i.e., with as little deliberation as possible. Have fun and play with it. Allow yourself to be free and honest. This is not a test of your artistic ability. If you don't want to draw, you may do a collage, once again choosing the first thing that suits your fancy. Allow it to be a drawing or a collage of free association. Give yourself permission to surprise yourself, if that is what your unconscious is trying to do. You do not have to be afraid of what emerges, as we only allow ourselves to see that which we are ready to look at. Take a risk. It can do you no harm, and it is possible that great good can come to you when you break through some of your denial.

Support Person

Draw a picture of your partner and your baby. Draw a picture, or do a collage, of yourself in relation to them. Include in the picture anything about pregnancy or parenthood that you find exciting, fearsome, of anxiety producing. Please read the mother's exercise and follow the same pattern of openness as is suggested to her.

After completing your drawing, continue to the next step of the exercise.

What are three things that you like about your drawing? What are three things that you don't like? What would you like to change about your drawing? Now make a list, as follows:

	Positive Feelings	Negative/Ambivalent Feelings
Marriage		
Pregnancy		
Labour		
Birthing		
Parenthood		
Breast Feeding		
Career		

Share your drawing and your feelings with someone who you can trust, and spend some time discussing these issues. Ask yourself, in order to feel happier in your daily life, how do you need to change your thinking, your attitudes, your beliefs, and your behavior (your feelings will follow) around the negative or ambivalent feelings you have listed. Take some time to do this during the first trimester and redo during the second and third trimester. Ask your partner and/or support person to do the same, and then spend some time during each trimester discussing your attitudes without being judgmental of either yourself or your partner. Remain open and curious.

In order to understand the Leclaire method better, let us look for a moment at a problem of a patient named Kathleen. Kathleen came into therapy when she was seventeen weeks pregnant. She had been experiencing severe nausea and vomiting which was beginning to subside. She had been raped when she was in college and was so shamed by the experience that she never discussed it with anyone in her family. Her husband had no knowledge of her horrible experience, either. It became imperative for her to discuss this horrific happening while she was pregnant. She felt guilty and dishonest, as through she had violated her marriage and wasn't deserving of real serenity and happiness! She felt that her husband rightly honored his mother more than he did Kathleen. After all, how could James respect her after she was brutally sexually violated. The damage was rather engraved upon her being. Through individual therapy and the Rape Crisis Center, Kathleen was able to let go of much of her negativity. Her relationship with her husband and her mother-in-law improved, and her relationship with herself and her baby became one of calm acceptance.

All good education brings us toward our ultimate goal in life: an ability to exercise all of the faculties we have been given. Thus, we need to train our minds, our bodies, and our spirits. If each mother accepts individual responsibility for herself, and along with that acceptance she takes the initiative to act, i.e., to be able to move toward a pregnancy and childbirth the way it was intended to be, she can experience a celebration of life. Kathleen, and many other women with whom I have worked, have participated with great courage and have embraced a wonderful feeling of freedom and accomplishment through the birthing process.

At the beginning of the 20th century when a woman experienced pain in childbirth she was rendered unconscious. Today it is becoming apparent that the more aware a woman is, the more comfortable she will be during childbirth. The more we take control of our bodies, our selves, and our lives, the less we shall suffer on every plane. Unconsciousness means loss of awareness, and loss of awareness means an inability to experience the great joy and miracle of childbirth.

❖ Chapter Two

Myths Surrounding Childbirth

Pavlov taught us that even the most pleasant of associations can be conditioned to become fearful if paired with an unpleasant or frightening stimulus.

In Western society childbirth has often been paired with horror stories of pain, puerperal fever, even death. The exaggeration, the creation of fear around childbirth, and the role of the father as a bumbling idiot have been perpetuated by the movie industry. It makes for great dramatic film footage and allows for maintenance of the following myths in our culture:

1. Childbirth is painful and unbearable.
   a. I have heard many firsthand stories from friends and relatives.
   b. I have seen the agony of the mother innumerable times on the movie screen.
2. Labor inevitably ends up as a stressful emergency.
   a. I have often seen a screaming, out-of-control woman being rushed on a stretcher through the corridors of a hospital to the delivery room (not a birthing room).
3. The mother, now in agony, finds it impossible to birth her own baby. It becomes imperative for the doctor to put her out of her misery and to subsequently deliver the baby for her.
4. Throughout all of this, the father remains helpless and ridiculous, a buffoon of sorts, adding the necessary comic relief to the heavy drama at hand.

Just as good education should bring us back to our original essence, so good culture should elevate our basic natures and purge it of the contamination of civilization. It seems that our Western culture has affected the natural function of our birthing. It has taken a relatively painless event, a beautiful miracle of life, and turned it into a period of anxiety, exhaustion, fear and pain.

Origin of Myths Surrounding Childbirth

The history of childbirth in European civilization has fostered the concept of pain and suffering as an essential component. A second grader, when asked the definition of history, said it is something that goes on and on and on. It is possible to stop this man-made idea of childbirth by reconnecting ourselves to the beauty and simplicity of childbirth that "indigenous" (natural) women have experienced for all time. These are the women who have not been historied by an imposing, negative culture. They expect an easy and unlabored childbirth, and that is what they receive. They are in accord with their own unaffected nature.

Relaxed childbirth conforms to the laws of nature. Hippocrates, the father of medicine who lived about 400 years before Christ, stressed prevention of complications through discipline in diet, exercise, and fresh air. He also concentrated on self-healing through attending to our own nature. He taught his students not to interfere with nature, to intervene only in case of emergency, to first do no harm, and not to administer any deadly drugs.

Aristotle (384-322 B.C.) recognized that the mind of the mother must be cared for during pregnancy. Soranus, the grand authority of obstetrics in Greece, wrote a treatise in 79 A.D. on obstetrics in which he emphasized the acknowledgement of the "women's feelings." Fear was not a normal occurrence during childbirth at that time. Today, however, we might say it is normal/usual for a woman to feel fear.

About 300 years after Christ, Soranus' treatise, and all other books on medicine that believed in the laws of nature, became a heinous crime against the Church; thus, these works were buried. Childbirth was seen as the result of a sin of the flesh, and to be forgiven, one had to suffer. No man, except a shepherd, was allowed to attend a birth. One German doctor who dressed up as a midwife was found out and burned at the stake.

There is a passage in the Bible — "I will greatly multiply thy sorrow and thy conception; in sorrow thou shalt bring forth children." This is a sorrow that was imposed upon Eve as she grieved for her children who would be born with original sin. Her sorrow was imposed upon her because she chose carnal pleasure. Her choice rendered her unable to have an immaculate conception and a virgin birth. Thus, this is a spiritual rendering of sorrow in the fashion of hell being the absence of the beatific vision. Can a child who is tainted with sin be born alive? Perhaps the Bible has taught women to fear childbirth, to fear the birth of a child born with original sin. Perhaps if a woman suffers during childbirth, she can expiate her child of his original sin. If she suffers enough, and he is expiated, then and only then can he be born healthy. After all, how can one who is in sin be unscathed, and healthy and beautiful, unless he is washed clean through his own penance or that of his mother?

In 1947 chloroform was discovered as an anesthesia and used for women in childbirth. But the Church disapproved of relieving the pain of women in childbirth.

Perhaps they felt the pain of childbirth had been imposed upon women for their spiritual blunders (or for Eve's spiritual blunder). Christianity teaches that God is love. A pregnant woman is like Eve, in that she has chosen the love of man over God. God did not give sexual pleasure to humanity. God gave free will, and man chose carnal pleasure. The God who said, "In sorrow thou shalt bring forth thy children" still wields His power in the birthing rooms. If this is a belief system that has been imposed upon us, let us face it. Let us accept our human choice and render it into the realm of consciousness. Let us not fragment ourselves by having our body do one thing, and our mind and spirit another.

Let us view pregnancy and childbirth as a time wherein we can again make the choice of the flesh or the spirit. The true lord within us is our harmonic spiritual essence — the god within integrates the mind and the body with itself, enabling each of us to become a whole person, to become a being true to our own nature. This connection to the godhead or "Mother Nature" allows each person to return to her own true being — her essence — her purification. Let us align ourselves to the celebration of our natural state.

In order to do this we need to deal with the obstructions our culture has placed in our path. It is pointless, a waste of time and unhealthy, for us to suffer because of the emotional beliefs others have imposed upon us. Our culture has been our truth. However, if we look to indigenous (natural) woman and to the animal world, we see a contradiction with our own. In the world of the indigenous woman and in the animal's world there is no apparent pain in birthing. The look of hard work on a mother's face can be confused with an affect of pain. The affect of a man or a woman having an orgasm can also appear to be painful. Does that mean that it is? Fear and pain as components of childbirth have entered our field of awareness. They have become an image of childbirth, a part of our reality. It would be helpful for us to take the seed of the indigenous woman's reality and recreate our own. It is time for our Western unconsciousness to progress into consciousness.

Since it became culturally important for a woman to suffer in childbirth, we have taken on the mechanical continuation of that act. The feeling of joy faded into the unconscious. We must awaken from this mechanized pattern and return ourselves to our source, to our level of comfort. We must dissociate from the myths of fear and pain and connect to our own individuation. We no longer have to keep negative concepts alive through our participation.

The Myth of the Virgin as it Relates to Bonding and Sexuality

Frequently, during postpartum women aren't very interested in their sexuality in the same way that a man is. One of the reasons is physical limitations, and another is cultural. These feelings of wanting to remain chaste oftentimes relate to another powerful myth that needs to be dispelled, the Myth of the Virgin.

In this myth, pleasure and pain are readily bonded. "That troublesome weariness with which all pregnant women are burdened; she alone did not experience who alone conceived without pleasure." In the Garden of Eden labour and pain did not exist. It was the choice of Adam and Eve that brought about our dissolute flesh, and marriage was born out of sin. After eating of the forbidden fruit, they became aware of their nakedness, they became aware of themselves. They were no longer in harmony with their environment. The observing ego now emerges and is omnipresent. Adam is no longer immortal: "from dust thou are and unto dust thou shalt return." And Eve is told, "I will greatly multiply thy sorrow and thy conception...and thy desire shall be to thy husband and he shall rule over thee" (Genesis 3:19, 16). It was here that pain and suffering were thrust upon woman.

A woman with original sin now could only birth a child with original sin. Only a virgin birth could eradicate the stain, the curse upon women, only chastity could sever the chain of sorrow and distress. Through chastity a woman could devote her life to God's work.

Since childbirth was woman's function, she was deemed more closely aligned to the evils of desire, of the flesh, and of sex. Thus, woman was more visibly evil than man. The only way a woman could redeem herself was to align with her spirituality, to align with Mary rather than with Eve.

A feast of the purification of the Virgin Mary was instituted in the Seventh century. This feast day also coincided with the pagan feast of light, when candles were held and carried on high in a procession in honor of the Virgin, and in order to exorcise all the spirits of the underworld that caused floods and famine and natural disasters. Thus, through Mary, preventive medicine became possible. Is it any wonder that in many cultures some form of the name Mary is given to all children, boys and girls alike? An association with the purity of Mary, the Virgin, is thought to dispel the taint of original sin. Thus, the blessing or churching/purification of a woman postpartum is still performed in many Catholic churches.

It is through the second Eve, Mary, that woman is redeemed. Mary is spotless, she is clean of original sin; she is also wise and fruitful. It is through the birth and death of her son that the world is saved. Mary does not suffer the burden of the fall; she is exempt from pain and suffering in childbirth and of bodily corruption in the grave. However, she did follow the natural law of lactation. Her milk was the life of the world. She fed the God who would redeem the world from the fall of Adam and Eve. When Mary died, she did not putrefy in the grave. She was assumed into heaven. Thus, she gave women a model to understand. The difference between Mary and other women is her immaculate conception, the virgin birth and her assumption into heaven.

She gave birth without pain, she suckled her infant, and she died, as we all shall do. What then are the consequences of Eve's sin? It seems the presence of the ego, dishonor in the eyes of men, and scapegoating by them, concupiscence, other earthly desires and putrefaction.

Mary's motherly concern for the partners in marriage becomes explicit in the story of the marriage in Cana, where she interceded with her son to turn the water into wine for the guests. The wine, the union of man and woman, is the lifeblood of the world after the fall. Her son obeys her, and blesses the union by turning the water into wine.

Much of this may sound like hocus-pocus or ridiculous philosophical thought. It may, in fact, be either or both of these. It may also be that the collective unconscious of our Western culture has passed these impressions on to us. If this is so, then we must deal with this issue. I believe in prevention, and I make the assumption that the myth of the Virgin is one that is all-pervasive in our society. Let us go on.

Jesus, being both divine and human, drank the pure milk of his mother's sinless breast, and also at the last supper, he drank of the wine as a symbol of the blood he was to shed for the redemption of woman and man.

The fertility of Mary, in the mythology, is a bond that ties her to the creativity of all women. The bond is not only the miracle of creation through motherhood, but also through the symbol of the milk that flows from woman's breast, the milk of life, the creative life-giving force that woman can share with the rest of humankind.

In the myth of the Virgin there is also included the dropping of her sash, her girdle, as she is assumed into heaven. It is an umbilical cord from heaven to earth, a symbol of her dualistic function. Through her giving to us a piece of her clothing she recognizes our materialism, our humanity, and yet she gives us a link to her, to our own spirituality through which we can have our pain eased.

A woman's work receives recognition only when its quality is much higher than that of a man's. If a woman's labour becomes joyous and spiritual, she on the one hand satisfies the Mother Church in that she aligns with the spirituality of Mary, and on the other hand she alters the role in which the patriarchy has placed her. Will this change in the quality of her childbirth give her more recognition or less?

Some of the pain and fear of childbirth may stem from the severance woman has experienced (on an unconscious level) from God/self due to the internalization of the myth of original sin. She holds within her for nine months, through the permissive will of God, a new soul, a new link. For forty weeks she bears a deep spiritual connection to God. At parturition she now must become separated from her child, from this new soul, from her link to God.

Our ego, our worldliness, is easily swayed from connecting with our spirituality. It is in childbirth that they are forced to approach each other beyond the usual spatial limit. The phenomenon of childbirth is the impetus that can eliminate the conflict.

Perhaps the bringing of the father to the fore during pregnancy reduces the woman's ancient burden. If she now outwardly shares her joy with the participating non-virginal male, her ascribed suffering can be diminished and even transcended. In so doing she is also being gracious in her allowance of the man's sharing in the resolution, the recognition and the new spiritual awareness. Here the mother now may redeem them both of the sin of Adam and Eve. Through altering of this history, and system, they can each move toward joy and greater liberation.

Religion is the ego's mechanism of regulating the spirit. The fault of religion is that the spirit as truth needs no regulating. It already encompasses all morality, all religion, all regulations. It is spiritual truth that is the ultimate goal of religion. One cannot regulate that which is regulation itself. One cannot attain reality by living only in a dream. The dream then becomes the mode of being, but not the reality one was seeking to find through the dream. One cannot be in a dream, and also in the state of reality consciousness. One also cannot be in a state of religion once one has found her soul/self, for religion is only a vehicle for attaining a spiritual reality, as the dream is the vehicle for psychic reality. Through knowledge of ourselves and our myths, we may evolve to a oneness of spirit, to that universal truth that lies within each one of us.

The universe/god, humanity, and the virgin/spirit are the singularity of the mind, the body and the soul/self.

It is through the union of the masculine (the perfect order and knowledge of the universe) with the self (the individualized human), our God consciousness, as well as with the feminine (the spiritual nurturer), that the turmoil of the individual can abate. It is here through this infinite bonding that the individual and the family can be renewed and restored.

This union is the wedded bliss we all so desperately long for; this is the rational/intuitive consciousness that accepts what religion excludes. In *A Brief History of Time*, Stephen Hawking discusses real and imaginary time, and then he writes:

...Scientific theory is just a mathematical model we make to describe our observations; it exists only in our minds, so it is meaningless to ask which is real, 'real' or 'imaginary' time? It is simply a matter of which is the most useful description.

The myths and models of our nature that add to our physical, mental and spiritual well-being are obviously more useful than those that do not. Through knowledge of ourselves and our myths we may evolve to a oneness of spirit, to that universal truth that lies within each one of us.

The following is an exercise to bring us closer to who we are, both as mothers and fathers:

1. Write out your goals around your designs for your life. Write them for now and for six months from now, and for one year from now. Make your goals measurable and easily attainable. Take baby steps rather than giant steps. It is easier to succeed this way.

    a.   Career
    b.   Motherhood
    c.   Fatherhood
    d.   Marriage
    e.   Creativity

f.   Spirituality
g.   Nutrition
h.   Exercise
i.   Play
j.   Social support
k.   Physical contact
l.   Mental stimulation

One of the things that I suggest around marriage is to include in your goals a period of bonding, to begin preferably during your pregnancy. Bonding is a time for mothers and fathers to be alone, to be there for each other, not talking about bills or criticisms, but rather caressing, massaging each other; it is a time to be together, alone, without the TV, without the phone. Start the pattern with a realistic amount of time — even five minutes, twice a week — and gradually build to a time that is acceptable to you both. It is very important to keep this up during the entire pregnancy and especially during the postpartum, specifically during the first three months after the birth. Be flexible and alter the amount of time as necessary. Be creative, especially after the baby arrives. Getting out of the house for a fifteen-minute walk may be the amount of time you will feel comfortable leaving the baby with a sitter. Do that for yourself. Most marital, including sexual, problems are both normal and transitory during pregnancy and the postpartum. When the baby is six to ten months old, all should be back to normal. A mother usually isn't physically recovered until three to six weeks postpartum. She isn't emotionally recovered until five to ten months after the birth. Take this into consideration when you are thinking about your sexual patterns, and make allowances.